Essential Oils for Anxiety

Essential Oil Recipes for
Anxiety
for Diffusers, Roller Bottles,
Inhalers & more.

Rica V. Gadi

ISBN: 9781792992346

http://eorecipes.net

This book is dedicated to all the strong people who are taking responsibility of your own well being and doing something to be better.

All my heartfelt gratitude to the following people: my mom Ruby Jane, you have made me everything I am today; my dad Nestor-- my eternal, my angel, and the source of my perseverance; Mommyling, my spiritual guide ; Ria & Joe, the true witnesses of my transformation and my foundation pillars; Ellie Jane, the sparkle of our eyes;

Juan, thanks for always encouraging me to push harder - you are my ONE; Rocco & Radha, my reason for everything.

The Love of my family and friends is the fountain of inspiration that never runs dry. Thank you for constantly inspiring me, motivating me, and loving me unconditionally.

This book will never be complete without the help of my trusted and talented friends the #NOWsuperstars and my #oilbularya friends

Blending Essential Oils to use for a very specific reason has become very popular in the recent years. There are several reasons why this is so. Blending EOs is basically about inhaling - as it has been proven that aromas have the ability to trigger feelings, emotions and personal memories.

With this in mind, it is obvious that everyone is unique when it comes to what triggers your senses. It all boils down to personal preference for the aroma to trigger what you want to unleash. Everyone is different and we all connect to the aroma differently, so what might work for one might not work for another person.

Of course, we also want the blend we personalize to be therapeutic. This is the best reason why to blend essential oils. We want the blend we create to help us with a very specific emotion or physical condition. As much as smelling good is important in a blend, it is more important that we blend oils that is not only pleasing to the smell but also produces the therapeutic effect we are after.

Then you have to think about contraindications. Making sure the blend you create is safe to use.

I suggest that before blending find out if the oils you are using is safe for a condition you may have example, if you are pregnant, or have specific allergies. Consult your physician prior to moving forward.

The recipes I have in this book is a compilation of what has proven to work and favored by hundreds of EO enthusiasts. It takes out the guesswork to get you started.

Again, we urge you to read the recipes and make sure that this is safe for you to try.

The book is very specific to a physical and emotional condition. There are several recipes here because you might want to rotate and you may like one and not the other. There is also a variety of application. Some of us prefer to diffuse, some to make roller bottles, and others to create sprays.

I hope you enjoy this compilation, feel free to use the notes section and jot down your fave blends. There is a wonderful world of EO blending - this is just the beginning.

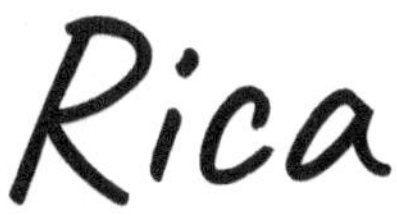

Anxiety is most definitely not random. It is not unknown and it is not an uncontrollable illness or disease that you can just get or develop, contract or inherit from your parents. Anxiety is caused by a certain type of behavior. This condition stems from a personal creation of the psychological, physiological or emotional anxious state when we behave in a certain way such as being fearful, worried and deep feelings of concern. Since everybody at any point gets worried, and is usually a normal behavior, these apprehensive feelings of Anxiety become a disorder when it starts to disrupts and interferes with a normal lifestyle.

Chronic Anxiety may have consequences and have serious effects to your physical health such as feelings of doom, depression, irritability, irregular heart rates, problems with breathing, panic attacks, migraines, loss or decreased libido, extreme fatigue and stomach/digestive problems.

It is time to see a physician when your anxiety is seriously affecting the way you live your everyday life. If extreme discomfort is felt for a long period of consecutive days, stopping you from doing the things you want or like to do, causing distances to your personal relationships with your family and friends or affecting the way you do your work due to Anxiety - it is best to seek medical attention.

Anxiety can become dangerous to your health when the stress starts to affect your body. Although stress is part of normal living, anxiety changes the way you look and live your life, That plus the stress it causes will definitely put a strain in your physical health and your immune system, causing inflammation and could lead to a chronic disease. It may affect the stability of your social, personal, emotional and professional life.

Essential Oils can help relieve these deep feelings of Anxiety by stimulating the receptors of smell through the nose, these receptors have the ability to send messages through the system to your nervous system. The brain controls the entire body and if the aroma can somehow send calming effects through the olfactory senses to the body , then it can also bring feelings of peace and calming.

Table of Contents

In today's world, emotional and mental unstableness has become a common issue in the society. This may consist of stress, nervousness, panic attacks, and others. Sometimes, however, it is normal to feel worried about some uncertainties but if this feeling gets unreasonable, a person might be already suffering from anxiety. Anxiety is pretty rampant nowadays. As a matter of fact, approximately 40% of adults and 10% of teens suffer from this mental illness in the US. Sufferers seldom get treatment through therapy and other form of medications but the current technology and modern medicine can help these individuals receive natural treatment through essential oils. Essential oils are known for their wondrous aroma but aside from that they are also beneficial for health. Luckily, there are essential oils for anxiety too. We aim to help the individuals who experience anxiety may it be mild or chronic, so listed below are the most suggested and recommended essential oils for anxiety.

Lavender Oil

Lavender oil comes first among all essential oils for anxiety. Lavender has sedative and calming properties which help an individual relax and reduce stress. It is one of the safest essential oils when the properties are properly attenuated. According to studies, people who suffer from sleep problems such as insomnia can use lavender oil as a remedy as it quickly passed to the bloodstream when inhaled. However, do not use this excessively as it can possibly act as a stimulant instead of giving a positive outcome on general well-being.

How do you use lavender as an essential oil for anxiety? You simply need to rub 2-3 drops of lavender oil on your palms and inhale for an immediate calming effect. To help you sleep, apply the oil to the soles, wrists, or palms. Another approach is combining lavender oil with jojoba or sweet almond (carrier oils). Once combined, the essential oil can be directly applied to the skin or added to your bath. You may also use the oil by adding it to a vaporizer or diffuser.

Ylang Ylang

Along with lavender, ylang ylang has sedative properties as well which help an individual in calming which may either be through inhalation, diffusion, or topical application. Aside from that, ylang ylang is best known for its capability in reducing stress, cortisol, and blood pressure while increasing the skin temperature which helps increase the functionality of the sympathetic nervous system.

Through topical application, simply rub a generous amount of ylang ylang essential oil on your palms and directly apply to wrists, neck, feet, and back to decrease the feeling of agitation and disturbance. However, according to users, it is best used in a diffuser or vaporizer as a great relief for anxiety and stress. You may not believe but it is even said to be an aphrodisiac.

Clary Sage

Clary sage is rich in linacyl acetate which was already proven in several studies to calm and relax the nervous system. It is best used as an anti-depressant and helps relieve chronic anxiety. This is also useful for women who suffer from hormonal shifts from menstruation and pregnancy. Clary sage is mildly sedative and also helps relieve hypertension. On another positive note, it uplifts your mood and it induces pleasure, self-esteem, confidence, and high spirit. Mainly because clary sage essential oil lowers the cortisol level which reduces stress and induces serotonin which increases mood stabilization.

At the comfort of your own home, simply use the oil in a diffuser for your anxiety and depression relief. As clary sage is amazingly fragrant, it invites you to a steam facial as well. As mentioned above, it also serves as a remedy for women when it comes to hormonal shifts and menstrual cramps. You only need a few drops of clary sage oil mixed with carrier oil, this time at least 10 ml of sweet almond oil and gently rub the mixture on your abdomen for several minutes. Another approach would be a clary sage mixture diluted in lukewarm water for a soothing bath which is also a great way in relieving cramps.

Vetiver

Vetiver was widely used in the ancient times to treat pain in the back and joints, as well as fever and scars. In the field of medicine, it also has potentials when used as an essential oil, particularly as an essential oil for anxiety. It is called "oil of tranquility" in Sri Lanka and India. Vetiver is a cooling oil which calms the mind. It reduces stress and alleviates anxiety level as well as depression, insomnia, and panic attacks. In the recent studies, vetiver was found to have sedative properties like the lavender which relieve inflammation of the nervous system. Vertiver essential oil can be used in reducing and calming the hyperactivity of children with ADHD and was revealed to have the most effective calming and ADHD-reducing effects.

To stabilize your emotions and to calm your mind, rub 3-5 drops of vetiver oil on your wrists, chests, and neck. It can be combined with a carrier oil like jojoba oil which leaves your skin moisturized and at the same time calming and relaxing your mind. You can also use a diffuser as the scent draws to the amygdala and attenuates its stress and anxiety response.

Chamomile

Like any other essential oils, chamomile is best known for its sedative properties and its wonderfully fragrant scent. Studies showed that chamomile helps individuals who suffer from mild or moderate anxiety disorder. Chamomile essential instills calmness in both the body and mind. It also alleviates stress and reduces anxiety while inducing sleep effectively. It was also revealed that it heals and reduces inflammation in the digestive tract. How does the digestive connect to anxiety and the nervous system? You may not be aware that there is a portion of our nervous system which can be found on intestines known as the enteric nervous system. Approximately 90% of serotonin is produced in the gut which helps in stabilizing your emotions and uplifting your mood. Disturbances in the digestive tract may affect your mood and may increase levels of anxiety. As such, chamomile relaxes the intestines and reduces anxiety and stress.

These chamomile benefits can be enjoyed by applying a generous amount directly applied to the skin or can be used in a humidifier. Basically the essential oils for anxiety can be used in multiple ways which again can be through inhalation, topical application, and diffusion.

As people developed anxiety rooted from various experiences, medications were also improved. Treatment from therapies evolved to natural treatments which include essential oils. While these oils smell wonderfully fragrant, they also give calmness both to your body and mind. As emphasized, these essential oils alleviate your stress and anxiety, and at the same time stabilize your mood and emotions. So if you are one of the sufferers, take the initiative to try and enjoy the benefits of essential oils for anxiety. No matter where you are, they could be of great help for your comfortableness and general well-being. .

It is also worth mentioning that the following oils are worth checking out for Migraines : **Jasmine, Frankincense, Valerian, Sweet Basil, Patchouli, Bergamot, Sweet Orange, Eucalyptus**

The Blending Process

These EOs are categorized by aromas, and EOs from the same group usually blend fantastically together.

- Floral – Lavender, Geranium, Jasmine
- Woodsy – Pine, Cedarwood
- Earthy – Vetiver, Patchouli
- Herbaceous – Marjoram, Rosemary, Basil
- Minty – Peppermint, Spearmint, Wintergreen
- Medicinal – Eucalyptus, Frankincense, Melaleuca
- Spicy – Pepper, Clove, Cinnamon
- Oriental – Ginger, Patchouli
- Citrus – Wild Orange, Lemon, Lime

Select oils that will give you with the health benefits you are looking to remedy. For increased energy choose: Grapefruit, Lemon, Orange, or Citrus. For Calming and Relaxation choose: Lavender, Cedarwood, or Chamomile. You are encouraged to experiment and play with your oils to see which blends work for you.

TIPS:

- Combine Floral EOs with Woodsy, Spicy and Citrus aromas
- Minty EOs with Woodsy, Earthy, Herbaceous and Citrus aromas
- Earthy EOs with Woodsy and Minty aromas
- Citrus EOs with Floral, Woodsy, Minty, Spicy and Oriental aromas

Diffuse

Diffusing Essential Oils is the safest method to enjoy Essential Oils without the risk of an allergic reaction.

Diffusing Essential Oils
Some Tidbits You Need To Know

Our sense of smell is one of our most powerful senses, and as you have noticed in your own experience that some scents affect your more positively in your minds than others. The body contains over 1,000 receptors for smell—way more receptors than for any of our other senses.

Diffusion Essential Oils means the process vaporizes oils into air by releasing tiny amounts into the air. Inhalation is totally safe and is super low risk. Chances of any EO rising to dangerous levels while diffusion is slim to none.

Diffusing Essential Oils around newborns, babies, young children, pregnant or nursing women, and pets should be done with caution. Read up on safety.

It is advisable that Diffusing Essential Oils for only about 15-30 minutes at a time to be most effective. NEVER leave your diffuser on overnight. Make sure your diffuser is filled with the right amount of water and you understand the operating directions.

While diffusing essential oils, be sure that your space has great ventilation. Crack a window open if the scent become to strong.

Never add Carrier Oils to your diffuser. This may cause your diffuser to malfunction. Clean your diffuser at least 3 times a week with warm water and natural soap to ensure the diffuser is well maintained and bacteria and mold does not accumulate.

Diffusing Essential Oils
Basic Guidelines

Just a few things you need to know and prepare before getting started Diffusing Essential Oils.

Things you need:
Ultrasonic Oil Diffuser
Essential Oils
Water

Just follow the number of drops in the recipe, drop on to an oil diffuser and fill the rest with water.

All diffusers are different and will have its own water minimum and maximum level. Read the diffuser instruction before use.

Ideally, it is best to diffuse for 15-30 minutes and turn off the diffuser. The effect should be good for at least 2-3 hours. Turn your diffuser back on after 3 hours to reinforce oil diffusing effects.

It is not advisable to use EO in humidifiers.These are not made to release EOS

Diffuser Recipes

Here's a thought for you:

You may be wondering how aroma can simply eliminate symptoms. There's a simple answer to this : Aroma is simply a by-product of diffusing. It's the added benefit but in reality the real benefit comes from the air we breathe and how the body easily absorbs the essential oils released in the air. It works 2 ways, not only does it improve the air quality you breath by disinfecting and eliminating pollutants it also allows your glands to absorb the healing elements of the EOs released in the air molecules,

So for here are a few recipes that can help you manage symptoms and actual issues regarding the matter :

5 Drops Sandalwood
1 Drop Neroli
1 Drop Roman Chamomile
1 Drop Lavender

----

4 Drops Lavender
2 Drops Lemon
2 Drops Ylang Ylang

----

3 Drops Orange
2 Drops Bergamot
2 Drops Lavender

----

3 Drops Frankincense
2 Drops Lavender
2 Drops Wild Orange

----

3 Drops Patchouli
2 Drops White Fir
2 Drops Lavender

----

4 Drops Lavender
2 Drops Rosemary

----

3 Drops Patchouli
3 Drops Bergamot

----

2 Drops Geranium
2 Drops Clary Sage
1 Drop Patchouli
1 Drop Ylang Ylang

----

2 Drops Cedarwood
2 Drops Wild Orange
1 Drop Ylang Ylang
1 Drop Patchouli

----

3 Drops Lavender
3 Drops Lime
3 Drops Mandarin

4 Drops Lavender
2 Drops Cedarwood
2 Drops Wild Orange
1 Drop Ylang Ylang

----

3 Drops Frankincense
2 Drops Copaiba

----

3 Drops Lavender
2 Drops Stress Away
2 Drops Frankincense

----

5 Drops Frankincense
5 Drops Stress Away

----

3 Drops Peppermint
5 Drops Lavender
2 Drops Stress Away

----

4 Drops Bergamont
5 Drops Frankincense

----

4 Drops Stress Away
4 Drops Orange

----

2 Drops Purification
3 Drops Lemon
3 Drops Orange

----

2 Drops Grapefruit
2 Drops Bergamot
2 Drops Lime
2 Drops Ginger
1 Drop Sandalwood

----

3 Drops Orange
3 Drops Patchouli

----

2 Drops Lavender
2 Drops Cedarwood
2 Drops Roman Chamomile

----

4 Drops Lavender
3 Drops Chamomile

----

2 Drops Vetiver
2 Drops Cedarwood

----

2 Drops Grounding Blend
2 Drops Lavender

----

1 Drop Lavender
1 Drop Sweet (Wild) Orange
1 Drop Cedarwood
1 Drop Frankincense

----

2 Drops Lavender
2 Drops Lime
1 Drop Spearmint

----

2 Drops Lavender
2 Drops Bergamot
1 Drop Frankincense
3 Drops Lavender
3 Drops Bergamot

----

3 Drops Peppermint
3 Drops Lemon
2 Drops Orange

----

4 Drops Lavender
2 Drops Lemon
2 Drops Ylang Ylang

----

4 Drops Lavender
3 Drops Chamomile

Roll

Essential Oil Roller Bottles is the easiest method to enjoy Essential Oils Anywhere and Whenever.

Blending Essential Oils in a Roller Bottle
Some Tidbits You Need To Know

Essential Oils are usually super concentrated and too hard to measure how much to actually put straight from the bottle.

Roller bottles are a way that you are able to create blends ready to use with the right dilution. It allows your EO to last longer.

It also makes it easier to apply exactly where you want to target without getting it all over the place.

It is handy and easy to carry in your purse, ready to use at any time you want to.

I like to apply EOs at the bottom of the feet for many reasons. Our feet have bigger pores than any other skin in our bodies. this means that they are able to suck in the therapeutic compounds in our blend into the bloodstream faster that any other parts of the body. Imagine comparing a normal straw to an oversized straw and how much more you can suck in with the latter. This is how the soles of our feet is compared to the rest of the skin in our bodies.

The skin on our feet is also less sensitive and is designed to withstand some abuse. The risk of having an irritation from EOS is less likely to happen when applied on the feet.

The feet don't have the glands that act as a barrier. Sebaceous glands are glands in our skin that produces an oily substance called Sebum, for the purpose of lubricating and waterproofing the skin. Since this is oil and if you put oil on top of oil, it can act as a barrier or it may slow down penetration.

The feet and palms of our hands are the only skin that don't have these, so it is ideal to apply Essential Oils to the feet for maximum penetration.

Now, it would be hard to apply oils directly and very mess, right? Roller bottles make it super easy and convenient to roll the EOs at the bottom of our feet.

Carrier Oils Info

Carrier oils are vegetable-based oils with their own healing properties that dilute essential oils used to help carry the EOs into the skin.

Essential oils are highly concentrated and could evaporate very quickly. The carrier oil is mixed with the essential oil so it could penetrate the skin before it actually evaporates. Although EOs are oils, it is actually not that oily. When mixed with a carrier oil, it allows you to have more of the essential oil into your skin without wasting EOS to evaporate, making the healing properties of the EO strong and more effective.

There are also Essential oils that are too strong to apply directly to the skin and may cause damage, so it is important to dilute them with a carrier oil.

Never add Carrier Oils to your diffuser. This may cause your diffuser to malfunction. Clean your diffuser at least 3 times a week with warm water and natural soap to ensure the diffuser is well maintained and bacteria and mold does not accumulate.

Carrier Oils

There are a lot of different carrier oils that you can use with EOs to dilute them in a roller bottle.

To name a few :

Almond Oil - moisturizing and stays liquid at room temperature. Do not use if you are allergic to nuts.

Apricot Kernel Oil - moisturizing and suitable for sensitive skin or kids. It is super gentle on the skin.

Avocado Oil - moisturizing and suitable for sensitive and damaged skin. Perfect for skin problems.Can be mixed with other carrier oils

Castor Oil - with antibacterial, antiviral and antifungal properties, use topically to eliminate pain and relieve skin irritation.

Coconut Oil - its antibacterial, antiviral and antifungal properties it is the best and most versatile for skin care. The skin absorbs this very quickly. It solidifies in room temp and may still have a slight coconut oil aroma in it - but you can get a fractionated coconut oil to eliminate the 2 challenges above.

Grapeseed Oil - not just for cooking but also great for topical application on the skin.

Jojoba Oil - one of my faves for skin care blends. This oil is the closest to our natural oil our skin produces to it is absorbed easily without being oily. Also amazing for massage oil blends.

Olive Oil - this is the oil for herb type oils. mostly used for cooking but can also be applied to the skin but would need to be blended with a carrier oil that is mild and absorb well with the skin.

Rosehip Seed Oil - super good for deep moisturizing or skin irritations. This oil has a high content of antioxidants and helps remedy dry, scarred and wounded skin.

Recommended Roller Bottle Dilution Guide

RECOMMENDED ROLL-ON BOTTLE DILUTION AMOUNTS

5 ml (1/6 oz.) Roll-on Bottle = ~100 drops (1tsp.)
10 ml (1/3 oz.) Roll-on Bottle = ~200 drops (2 tsp.)
30 ml. (1 oz.) Roll-on Bottle = ~600 drops (6 tsp.)

Roll-on Size	5 ml	10 ml	30 ml	Add EO drops to roll-on, then fill with carrier oil.	Dilution Percentage
Essential Oil Drops	1	2	6	1%	
	2	4	12	2%	
	3	6	18	3%	
	5	10	30	5%	
	10	20	60	10%	
	20	40	120	20%	
	25	50	150	25%	
	50	100	300	50%	

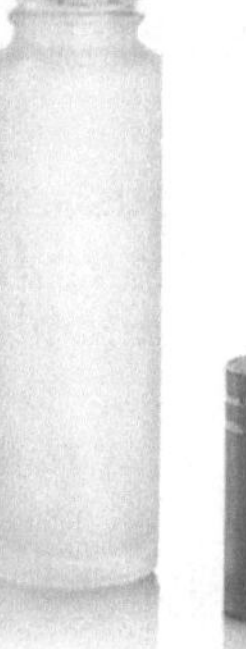
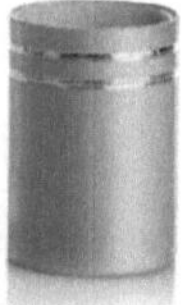

General Guidelines:
Birth to 12 months = .3-.5% dilution
1-5 years = 1.5-3% dilution
6-11 years = 1.5-5% dilution
12-17 years = 1.5-20% dilution
18 years and older = 1.5% dilution-Neat (no dilution)
Elderly or Sensitive Skin = 1-3% dilution
Daily Use = 2-5% dilution
Short Term Use = 10-25% dilution
Local Skin or Systemic Issues = 50% dilution-Neat

These are general guidelines suggestions--not absolute rules--based on traditional aromatheraphy practice.
(Kurt Schnaubelt PhD, Valerie Worwood, Robert Tisserand)

Dilution Basics:

How much you dilute your EO depends on different factors such as weight, sensitivity, health conditions, EOs that are blended in or how long that blend has been used for. There is never an absolute dilution rule, it is you who knows about your level and tolerance. I feel that it is best to start with a higher dilution percentage and increase EO drops over time.

To make sure your EO is safe, make sure that the oils you use are therapeutic grade and do your research on the source and extraction methods used to produce the oils.

Roller Bottle Blending Order

I normally just start with dropping the drops of oils into the **10mL roller bottle**, then adding the carrier oil up until the shoulder of the bottle. Capping the bottle off with the roller and the bottle cap. Instead of shaking the bottle, i like to roll the bottle between my palms first for a minute or 2 for blending, then finishing it off with a few shakes.

NOTE: All recipes in this book is for a 10mL Roller Bottle. If you have a bigger or smaller roller bottle, adjust the number of EO drops based on the size of your bottle.

Roller Bottle Recipes

2 drops Frankincense
2 drops Marjoram
3 drops Geranium
3 drops Clary sage
2 drops Orange

----

3 drops Wild Orange
3 drops Frankincense
3 drops Cinnamon

----

3 drops Inner Child
3 drops Grounding
3 drops Present Time
5 drops Valor or Valor II

----

4 drops Harmony
4 drops Forgiveness
4 drops Release
4 drops Lavender

----

4 drops Clary Sage
2 drops Fennel
4 drops Lavender
2 drops Geranium
2 drops Peppermint

----

5 drops Wild Orange
5 drops Frankincense
3 drops Cedar Wood
3 drops Lavender

----

5 drops Frankincense
3 drops Melissa
3 drops Patchouli

----

1 drops Patchouli
1 drops Vetiver
1 drops Lime
5 drops Balance
5 drops Lavender

----

6 drops Idaho Blue Spruce
6 drops Hong Kuai

----

4 drops Joy
3 drops Frankincense
3 drops Orange

----

4 drops Lavender
3 drops Clary sage
2 drops Ylang Ylang
1 drops Marjoram

----

5 drops Valor
4 drops Frankincense
4 drops Lavender
4 drops Cedarwood

----

2 drops White Angelica
2 drops Bergamot
2 drops Valor
2 drops Orange
1 drops Citrus Fresh

----

10 drops Lemon
4 drops Eucalyptus Radiata
3 drops Peppermint
1 drop Cinnamon

----

2 drops Patchouli
2 drops Elevation
2 drops Cedarwood
2 drops Balance
2 drops Basil
2 drops Vetiver

3 drops Black Pepper
3 drops Lime
3 drops Wild Orange
3 drops Frankincense

----

4 drops Bergamot
3 drops Wild Orange
2 drops Geranium
2 drops White Fir

----

7 drops Eucalyptus
5 drops Rosemary
3 drops Grapefruit

----

3 drops Spruce
3 drops Cedarwood
2 drops Juniper Berry
2 drops White Fir

----

4 drops Lavender
3 drops Lemon
2 drops Rosemary
1 drop Cinnamon

Bonus Recipes

Pain Relief Massage Oil Favorite

60mL Jojoba Oil (cold pressed)
8 drops Lavender
8 drops Peppermint
15 drops Frankincense

Pain Relief Massage Oil Secret

14 drops Frankincense
10 drops Sweet Orange
8 drops Turmeric
30mL Sweet Almond Oil

Pain Relief Bath Soak Blend

10 drops Frankincense
5 drops Lavender
5 drops Bergamot
1 cup Full-Cream/ Full-Fat Milk

Pain Relief Bath Salt Blend

1 cup Epsom Salt
¼ cup Dead Sea Salt
¼ cup Baking Soda
8-10 drops Essential Oils
(use any ingredient above or single oils)

Inhale

Essential Oil Inhalers are the most convenient way to enjoy Essential Oils Anywhere and Whenever.

Essential Oil Inhalers give you quick and easy access to the vast therapeutic benefits of essential oils.

Blending Essential Oils in an Inhaler
Some Tidbits You Need To Know

EO Inhalers or aroma sticks are compact tubes, with a cotton wick inside and a protective cover, to lock the aroma within.

Your preferred blend of essential oils is absorbed by the cotton wick, and safely enclosed in a tube that that fits inside of the cover. The cover is easily removed for access to the tube to breathe in the aroma. Usually lasts about 3 months, depending on the oil blend used.

I absolutely love these because they encourage me to take a moment during super stressful moments, and just breathe.

It is in times of stress when our breathing patterns often change and taking deep breaths promote a feeling of calm and inner peace. Breath work combined with visualization plus a relaxing inhaler, can offer relief to symptoms of stress and help your body to come back to the state of homeostasis.

Aroma Sticks can be carried in your tiny purse, even compact enough to fit in your pocket. You can enjoy your favorite EOs anywhere and you can use them with discretion.

I love diffusing, and do all the time but not everyone in my space may enjoy the scents I enjoy or they may not benefit from the therapeutic benefits of the EOs I am diffusing - so the inhaler is one way to not only enjoy my choice of blends but to keep in personal not affecting everyone else around me.

Inhalers not only benefits me but also keep those around me safe in case the oils I want to blend may pose a risk to those around me who may have health issue not advised to be exposed to my choice EOs/

When making Aroma Sticks, You may use your chosen EOs at 100% Concentration.

Inhaler Basic Guidelines

Breathe in slow and deep to absorb the EO molecules directly into your olfactory system.

Inhalers are super easy to use. You just remove the cap and inhale from the inhaler tube, count 1 to 5 slowly as you inhale. The EO molecules get drawn into our bloodstream through our nasal cavity and gets delivered throughout our entire body.

Simple to use, easy to cary, portable and compact. You never have to be without your favorite blends, ever.

Inhaler Blending Basics

Inhalers are super easy and simple to make.

All you need is an inhaler set which consist of the following:

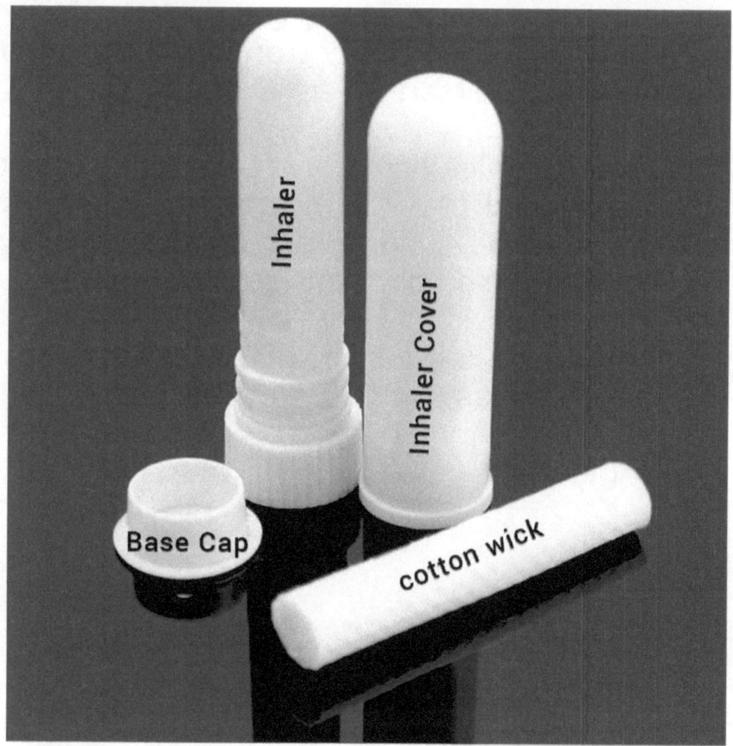

Inhaler, Inhaler Cover, Base Cap and Cotton Wick.

You will need your Essential Oils.

I like to use a pipette for precision and a small petri dish so I can see the oil.

Blending is super easy, just combine the drops and swirl it around in the petri dish and when you are satisfied you can go ahead and drop the cotton wick to absorb all the oil in the dish.

Once the wick is ready you can drop it in the inhaler and cap the bottom with the Base Cap. I usually like to secure the cover with the inhaler so I don't have to do it later.

I usually us 15-20 drops of EO total in a recipe and it can last up to 3 months. Some recipes will need more but on average it is in this range.

Inhaler Recipes

5 drops of Wild Orange
5 drops of Bergamot
5 drops of Sandalwood
5 drops of Ylang Ylang

----

10 drops of Vetiver
6 drops of Sandalwood or Cedarwood
5 drops of Ylang Ylang

----

4 drops of Ylang Ylang
7 drops of Orange
4 drops of Lavender

----

6 drops of Lemon
2 drops of Basil
2 drops of Rosemary
2 drops of Frankincense

----

6 drops of Lavender
3 drops of Lemon
3 drops of Ylang Ylang

----

10 drops of Roman Chamomile
5 drops of Lavender
3 drops of Vetiver

----

10 drops of Palmarosa
5 drops of Geranium
5 drops of Lavender

----

4 drops Lavender
4 drops Orange
4 drops Frankincense
3 drops Cedarwood

----

6 drops Lavender
5 drops Lime
4 drops Spearmint

----

8 drops of Lavender
4 drops of Roman Chamomile

----

5 drops of Frankincense
4 drops of Ylang Ylang
3 drops of Sandalwood
3 drops of Patchouli

----

6 drops of Tangerine
4 drops of Juniper
3 drops of Bergamot
2 drops of Clary Sage

----

4 drops of Cinnamon
4 drops of Balsam Fir
2 drops of Peppermint
5 drops of Orange

----

4 drops of Dill
3 drops of Fennel
4 drops of Lavender
4 drops of Lemongrass

----

4 drops of Grapefruit
3 drops of Spruce
3 drops of Geranium
1 drop of Palmarosa

----

10 drops of Ylang Ylang
6 drops of Lavender
4 drops of Patchouli

----

12 drops of Bergamot
6 drops of Lavender
2 drops of Frankincense

<u>Book Ordering</u>

To order your copy / copies of
Essential Oils for Anxiety

please visit: **EOrecipes.net**

You can also check out other titles available.

Bulk Pricing and
Affiliate Programs Available